Air Fryer Toaster Oven Best Recipes

Get In Shape And Lose Weight With Tasty And Affordable Recipes For Beginners

Eva Morris

TABLE OF CONTENT

Sweet Potatoes With Tofu..8

Gold Ravioli.. 10

Mediterranean Air Fried Veggies............................ 12

Super Veg Rolls... 14

Rice And Eggplant Bowl...................................... 16

Potatoes With Zucchinis...................................... 18

Blistered Shishito Peppers................................... 20

Mascarpone Mushrooms...................................... 23

Air Fried Asparagus...25

Cheesy Macaroni Balls.. 26

Crispy Chickpeas.. 29

Fig, Chickpea, And Arugula Salad........................ 30

Sriracha Golden Cauliflower................................33

Roasted Apple Sweet Potatoes............................35

Cheesy Broccoli Casserole................................... 37

Parmesan Brussels Sprouts.................................. 40

Garlicky Cauliflower Florets................................ 42

Flavors Green Beans..44

Potato Casserole... 46

Zucchini Egg Bake.. 49

Balsamic Baked Mushrooms................................. 51

Curried Cauliflower.. 53

Carnitas.. 55

Greek Lamb Meatballs... 58

Sesame Ginger Pork Meatballs..................................... 60

Chili Beef Skewers.. 63

Chipotle Pork Tenderloin Roast.................................... 65

Italian Ribeye Steak.. 67

Lamb Gyro... 69

Sausage Hot Pot.. 72

- 2 tablespoons unsalted butter................. 72
- ¼ teaspoon kosher salt........................... 72
- ¼ teaspoon black pepper......................... 72
- 5 sprigs thyme....................................... 72
- 1 whole onion, sliced.............................. 72
- 12 cremini mushrooms, sliced................. 72
- ½ cup red wine...................................... 72
- 1 cup beef broth..................................... 72
- 1 tablespoon parsley, chopped................ 72

Roast Beef.. 75

- 1 round roast (3 pounds)........................ 75
- ½ teaspoon paprika................................ 75
- ½ teaspoon garlic powder........................ 75
- ½ teaspoon black pepper......................... 75
- 1 tablespoon olive oil............................. 75
- 1 tablespoon Dijon mustard.................... 75

Air Fried Brussels Sprouts.. 77

Simple Buffalo Cauliflower...80

Crispy Jicama Fries...82

Zucchini Balls..84

Cheesy Potatoes And Asparagus 10..87

Saltine Wax Beans..89

Potato With Creamy Cheese...91

Easy Rosemary Green Beans...93

Garlic Eggplant Slices...95

Herbed Radishes..97

Sesame Taj Tofu..99

Chili Fingerling Potatoes..101

Sweet And Sour Tofu..103

Easy Potato Croquettes...105

this book has been derived from various sources. Please consult a licensed professional before attempting any techniques outlined in this book.

By reading this document, the reader agrees that under no circumstances is the author responsible for any losses, direct or indirect, which are incurred as a result of the use of information contained within this document, including, but not limited to, — errors, omissions, or inaccuracies.

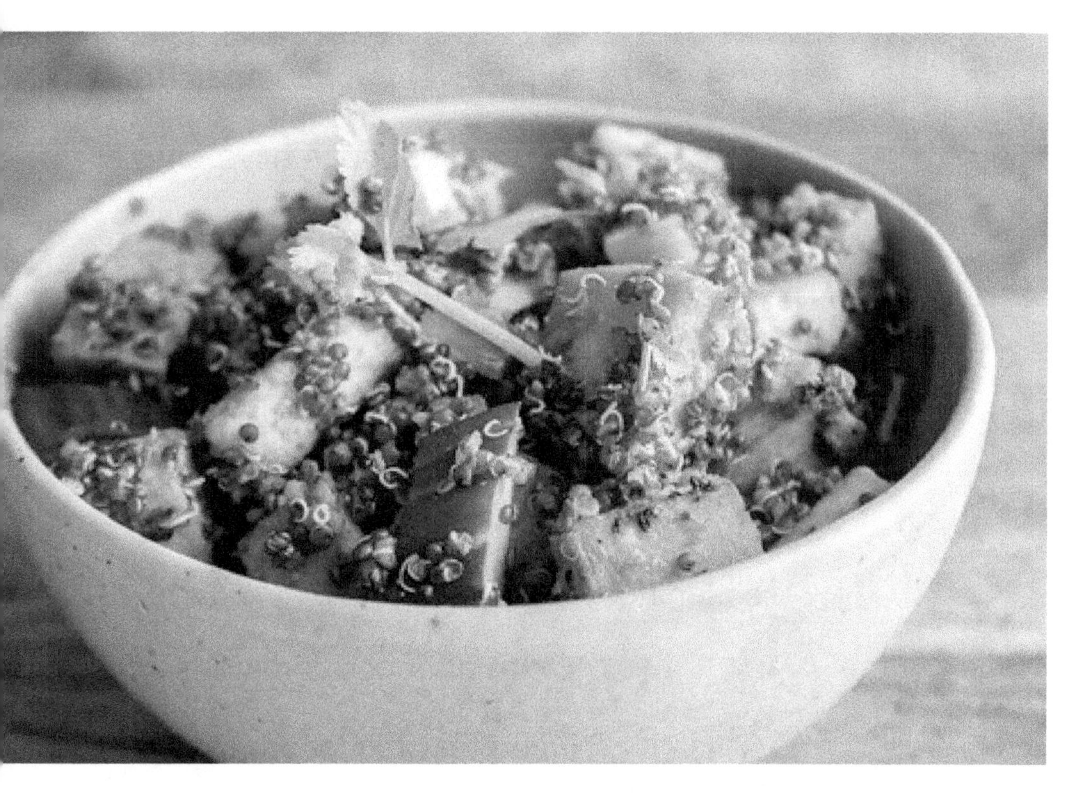

Sweet Potatoes With Tofu

Preparation Time: 15minutes

Cooking Time: 35 minutes

Serving: 8

Ingredients:

- Eight sweet potatoes, scrubbed
- Two tablespoons olive oil
- One large onion, chopped
- Two green chilies, deseeded and chopped
- 8 ounces (227 g) tofu, crumbled
- Two tablespoons Cajun seasoning
- 1 cup chopped tomatoes
- One can of kidney beans, drained and rinsed
- Salt and ground black pepper, to taste

Directions:

1. Press Start/Cancel. Preheat the air fryer oven to 400ºF (204ºC).

2. With a knife, pierce the skin of the sweet potatoes and transfer to the fry basket. Insert the fry basket at mid position. Select Air Fry, Convection, and set time to 30 minutes, or until soft.

3. Remove from the air fryer oven, halve each potato, and set to one side.

4. Over medium heat, fry the onions and chilies in the olive oil in a skillet for 2 minutes until fragrant.

5. Add the tofu and Cajun seasoning and air fry for a further 3 minutes before incorporating the kidney beans and tomatoes. Sprinkle some salt and pepper as desire.

6. Top each sweet potato halves with a spoonful of the tofu mixture and serve.

Gold Ravioli

Preparation Time: 10minutes

Cooking Time: 6 minutes

Serving: 4

Ingredients:

- ½ cup panko bread crumbs
- Two teaspoons nutritional yeast
- One teaspoon dried basil
- One teaspoon dried oregano
- One teaspoon garlic powder
- Salt and ground black pepper, to taste
- ¼ cup aquafaba
- 8 ounces (227 g) ravioli
- Cooking spray

Directions:

1. Cover the fry basket with aluminum foil and coat with a light brushing of oil.

2. Press Start/Cancel. Preheat the air fryer oven to 400ºF (204ºC). Combine the panko bread crumbs, nutritional yeast, basil, oregano, and garlic powder. Sprinkle with salt and pepper to taste.

3. Put the aquafaba in a separate bowl. Dip the ravioli in the aquafaba before coating it in the panko mixture. Spritz with cooking spray and transfer to the fry basket. Insert the fry basket at mid position.

4. Select Air Fry, Convection, and set time to 6 minutes. Shake the fry basket halfway.

5. Serve hot.

Mediterranean Air Fried Veggies

Preparation Time: 10minutes

Cooking Time: 6 minutes

Serving: 4

Ingredients:

- One large zucchini, sliced
- 1 cup cherry tomatoes, halved
- One parsnip, sliced
- One green pepper, sliced
- One carrot, sliced
- One teaspoon mixed herbs
- One teaspoon mustard
- One teaspoon garlic purée
- Six tablespoons olive oil
- Salt and ground black pepper, to taste

Directions:

1. Press Start/Cancel. Preheat the air fryer oven to 400ºF (204ºC).

2. Combine all the ingredients in a bowl, making sure to coat the vegetables well.

3. Transfer to the fry basket and insert the fry basket at mid position. Select Air Fry, Convection, and set time to 6 minutes, ensuring the vegetables are tender and browned.

4. Serve immediately.

Super Veg Rolls

Preparation Time: 20minutes

Cooking Time: 10 minutes

Serving: 6

Ingredients:

- Two potatoes, mashed
- ¼ cup peas
- ¼ cup mashed carrots
- One small cabbage, sliced
- ¼ cups beans
- Two tablespoons sweet corn
- One small onion, chopped
- ½ cup bread crumbs
- One packet spring roll sheets
- ½ cup cornstarch slurry

Directions:

1. Press Start/Cancel. Preheat the air fryer oven to 390°F (199°C).

2. Boil all the vegetables in water over low heat. Rinse and allow drying.

3. Unroll the spring roll sheets and spoon equal amounts of vegetables onto the center of each one. Fold into spring rolls and coat each one with the slurry and bread crumbs. Transfer to the fry basket.

4. Insert the fry basket at mid position. Select Air Fry, Convection, and set time to 10 minutes.

5. Serve warm.

Rice And Eggplant Bowl

Preparation Time: 15minutes

Cooking Time: 10 minutes

Serving: 4

Ingredients:

- ¼ cup sliced cucumber

- One teaspoon salt

- One tablespoon sugar

- Seven tablespoons Japanese rice vinegar

- Three medium eggplants, sliced

- Three tablespoons sweet white miso paste

- One tablespoon miring rice wine

- 4 cups cooked sushi rice

- Four spring onions

- One tablespoon toasted sesame seeds

Directions:

1. Coat the cucumber slices with the rice wine vinegar, salt, and sugar.

2. Put a dish on top of the bowl to weigh it down thoroughly.

3. In a bowl, mix the eggplants, miring rice wine, and miso paste. Allow marinating for half an hour.

4. Press Start/Cancel. Preheat the air fryer oven to 400ºF (204ºC).

5. Put the eggplant slices in the fry basket and insert the fry basket at mid position. Select Air Fry, Convection, and set time to 10 minutes.

6. Fill the bottom of a serving bowl with rice and top with the eggplants and pickled cucumbers.

7. Add the spring onions and sesame seeds for garnish. Serve immediately.

Potatoes With Zucchinis

Preparation Time: 10minutes

Cooking Time: 45 minutes

Serving: 4

Ingredients:

- Two potatoes, peeled and cubed
- Four carrots, cut into chunks
- One head broccoli, cut into florets
- Four zucchinis, sliced thickly
- Salt and ground black pepper, to taste
- ¼ cup olive oil
- One tablespoon dry onion powder

Directions:

1. Press Start/Cancel. Preheat the air fryer oven to 400ºF (204ºC).

2. In a baking dish, add all the ingredients and combine well. Insert at a low position.

3. Select Bake, Convection, and set time to 45 minutes, ensuring the vegetables are soft and the sides have browned before serving.

Blistered Shishito Peppers

Preparation Time: 10minutes

Cooking Time: 6 minutes

Serving: 4

Ingredients:

Dipping Sauce:

- 1 cup sour cream

- Two tablespoons fresh lemon juice

- One clove garlic, minced

- One green onion (white and green parts), finely chopped

- Peppers:

- 8 ounces (227 g) shishito peppers

- One tablespoon vegetable oil

- One teaspoon toasted sesame oil

- Kosher salt and black pepper, to taste

- •   ¼ to ½ teaspoon red pepper flakes

- •   ½ teaspoon toasted sesame seeds

Directions:

1. In a small bowl, stir all the ingredients for the dipping sauce to combine. Cover and refrigerate until serving time.

2. Press Start/Cancel. Preheat the air fryer oven to 400ºF (204ºC).

3. Toss the peppers with the vegetable oil. Then put the peppers in the fry basket.

4. Insert the fry basket at mid position. Select Air Fry, Convection, and set time to 6 minutes or until peppers are lightly charred in spots, stirring the peppers halfway through the cooking time.

5. Transfer the peppers to a serving bowl.

6. Drizzle with the sesame oil and toss to coat —season with salt and pepper.

7. Sprinkle with the red pepper and sesame seeds and toss again.

8. Serve immediately with the dipping sauce.

Mascarpone Mushrooms

Preparation Time: 10minutes

Cooking Time: 15 minutes

Serving: 4

Ingredients:

- Vegetable oil spray

- 4 cups sliced mushrooms

- One medium yellow onion, chopped

- Two cloves garlic, minced

- ¼ cup heavy whipping cream or half-and-half

- 8 ounces (227 g) mascarpone cheese

- One teaspoon dried thyme

- One teaspoon kosher salt

- One teaspoon black pepper

- ½ teaspoon red pepper flakes

- 4 cups cooked konjac noodles, for serving

- • ½ cup grated Parmesan cheese

Directions:

1. Press Start/Cancel. Preheat the air fryer oven to 350ºF (177ºC). Spray a heatproof pan with vegetable oil spray.

2. In a medium bowl, combine the mushrooms, onion, garlic, cream, mascarpone, thyme, salt, black pepper, and red pepper flakes. Stir to combine. Transfer the mixture to the prepared pan.

3. Put the pan in the fry basket. Insert at a low position. Select Bake, Convection, and set time to 15 minutes, stirring halfway through the baking time.

4. Divide the pasta among four shallow bowls. Spoon the mushroom mixture evenly over the pasta. Sprinkle with Parmesan cheese and serve.

Vegetable Sides

Air Fried Asparagus

Preparation Time: 5minutes

Cooking Time: 5 minutes

Serving: 4

Ingredients:

- 1 pound (454 g) fresh asparagus spears, trimmed
- One tablespoon olive oil
- Salt and ground black pepper, to taste

Directions:

1. Press Start/Cancel. Preheat the air fryer oven to 375ºF (191ºC).

2. Combine all the ingredients and transfer them to the fry basket. Insert the fry basket at mid position.

3. Select Air Fry, Convection, and set time to 5 minutes, or until soft.

4. Serve hot.

Cheesy Macaroni Balls

Preparation Time: 10minutes

Cooking Time: 10 minutes

Serving: 2

Ingredients:

- 2 cups leftover macaroni
- 1 cup shredded Cheddar cheese
- ½ cup flour
- 1 cup bread crumbs
- Three large eggs
- 1 cup milk
- ½ teaspoon salt
- ¼ teaspoon black pepper

Directions:

1. Press Start/Cancel. Preheat the air fryer oven to 365ºF (185ºC).

2. In a bowl, combine the leftover macaroni and shredded cheese.

3. Pour the flour into a separate bowl. Put the bread crumbs in a third bowl. Finally, in a fourth bowl, mix the eggs and milk with a whisk.

4. With an ice-cream scoop, create balls from the macaroni mixture. Coat them the flour, then in the egg mixture, and lastly in the bread crumbs.

5. Arrange the balls in the fry basket and insert the fry basket at mid position. Select Air Fry, Convection, and set time to 10 minutes, giving them an occasional stir. Ensure they crisp up nicely.

6. Serve hot.

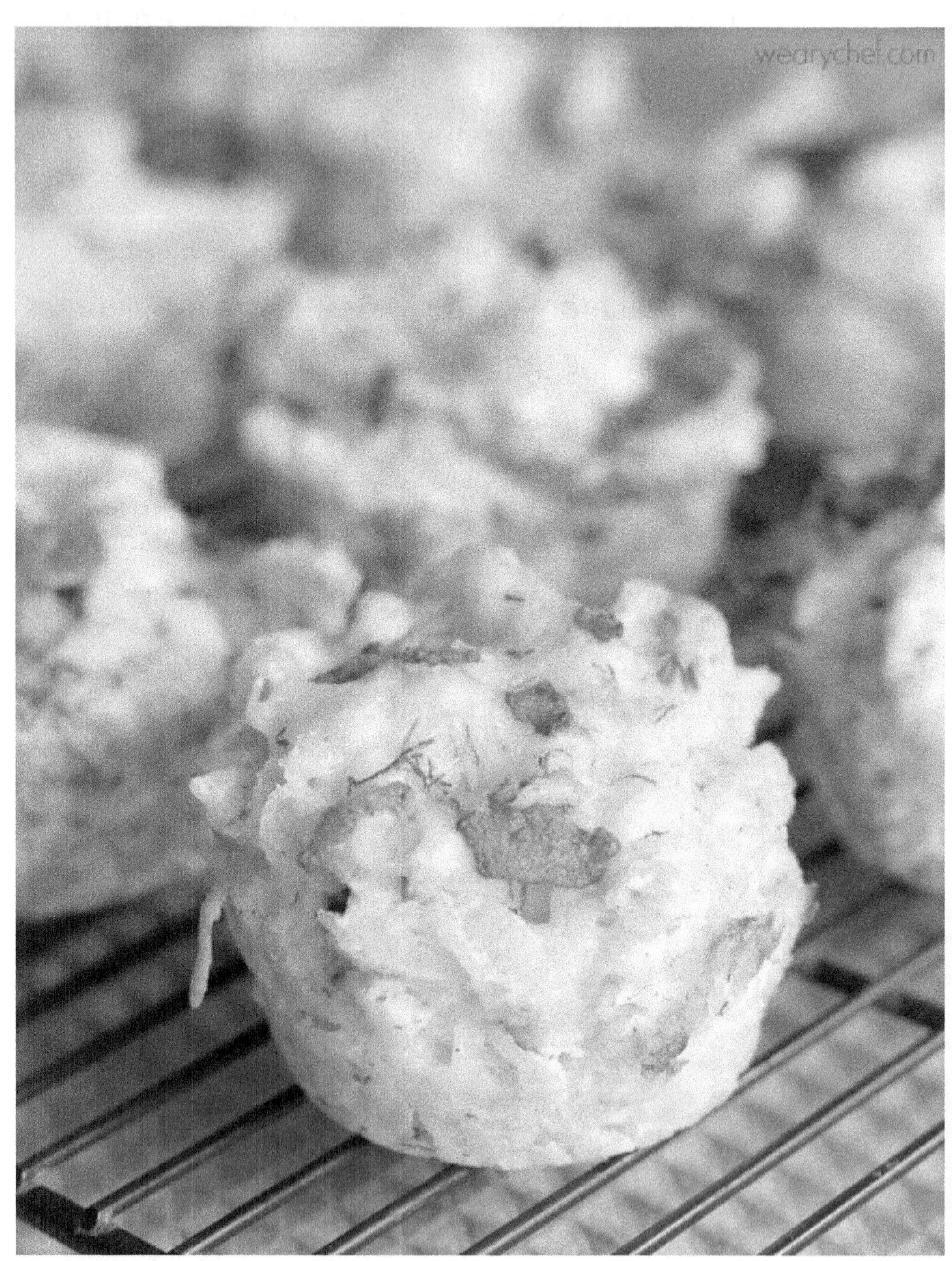

Crispy Chickpeas

Preparation Time: 5minutes

Cooking Time: 15 minutes

Serving: 4

Ingredients:

- 1 (15-ounces / 425-g) canned chickpeas, drained but not rinsed

- Two tablespoons olive oil

- One teaspoon salt

- Two tablespoons lemon juice

Directions:

1. Press Start/Cancel. Preheat the air fryer oven to 400ºF (204ºC).

2. Combine all the ingredients into a bowl. Then transfer this to the fry basket. Insert the fry basket at mid position.

3. Select Air Fry, Convection, and set time to 15 minutes, ensuring the chickpeas become nice and crispy.

4. Serve immediately.

Fig, Chickpea, And Arugula Salad

Preparation Time: 15minutes

Cooking Time: 20minutes

Serving: 4

Ingredients:

- Eight fresh figs halved

- 1½ cups cooked chickpeas

- One teaspoon crushed roasted cumin seeds

- Four tablespoons balsamic vinegar

- Two tablespoons extra-virgin olive oil, plus more for greasing

- Salt and ground black pepper, to taste

- 3 cups arugula rocket, washed and dried

Directions:

1. Press Start/Cancel. Preheat the air fryer oven to 375ºF (191ºC).

2. Cover the fry basket with aluminum foil and grease lightly with oil. Put the figs in the fry basket and insert the fry basket at mid position. Select Air Fry, Convection, and set time to 10 minutes.

3. In a bowl, combine the chickpeas and cumin seeds.

4. Remove the air fried figs from the air fryer oven and replace it with the chickpeas. Air fry for 10 minutes. Leave to cool.

5. In the meantime, prepare the dressing. Mix the balsamic vinegar, olive oil, salt, and pepper.

6. In a salad bowl, combine the arugula rocket with the cooled figs and chickpeas.

7. Toss with the sauce and serve.

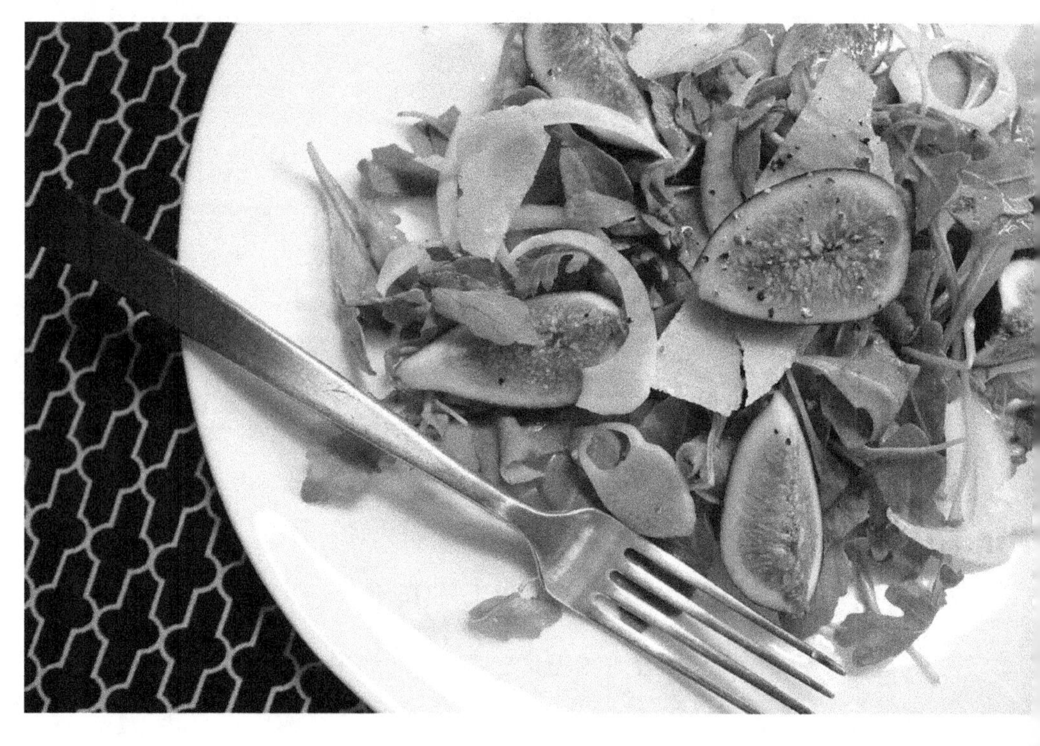

Sriracha Golden Cauliflower

Preparation Time: 5minutes

Cooking Time: 17 minutes

Serving: 4

Ingredients:

- ¼ cup vegan butter, melted
- ¼ cup sriracha sauce
- 4 cups cauliflower florets
- 1 cup bread crumbs
- One teaspoon salt

Directions:

1. Press Start/Cancel. Preheat the air fryer oven to 375ºF (191ºC).

2. Mix the sriracha and vegan butter in a bowl and pour this mixture over the cauliflower, taking care to cover each floret entirely.

3. In a separate bowl, combine the bread crumbs and salt.

4. Dip the cauliflower florets in the bread crumbs, coating each one well. Transfer to the fry basket. Insert the fry basket at mid position.

5. Select Air Fry, Convection, and set time to 17 minutes.

6. Serve hot.

Roasted Apple Sweet Potatoes

Preparation Time: 5 minutes

Cooking Time: 30 minutes

Serve: 2

Ingredients:

- Two large sweet potatoes, diced
- 2 tsp. cinnamon
- Two large green apples, diced
- 2 tbsp. maple syrup
- 1 tbsp. olive oil

Directions:

1. In a large bowl, add sweet potatoes, oil, cinnamon, and apples and toss well.

2. Spread sweet potatoes mixture onto the cooking pan.

3. Select bake mode and set the Omni to 400 F for 30 minutes once the oven beeps, place the cooking pan into the oven.

4. Drizzle with maple syrup and serve.

Nutrition:

Calories 352

Fat 7.6 g

Carbohydrates 74 g

Sugar 35.7 g

Protein 2.2 g

Cholesterol 0 mg

Cheesy Broccoli Casserole

Preparation Time: 5 minutes

Cooking Time: 30 minutes

Serve: 6

Ingredients:

- 16 oz. frozen broccoli florets, defrosted and drained

- 1/2 tsp. onion powder

- 10.5 oz. can cream of mushroom soup

- 1 cup cheddar cheese, shredded

- 1/3 cup unsweetened almond milk

For topping:

- 1 tbsp. butter, melted

- 1/2 cup cracker crumbs

Directions:

1. Add all ingredients except topping ingredients into the casserole dish.

2. In a small bowl, mix cracker crumbs and melted butter and sprinkle over the casserole dish mixture.

3. Select bake mode and set the Omni to 350 F for 30 minutes once the oven beeps, place the casserole dish into the oven.

4. Serve and enjoy.

Nutrition:

Calories 193

Fat 12.9 g

Carbohydrates 10.5 g

Sugar 2.4 g

Protein 6.9 g

Cholesterol 27 mg

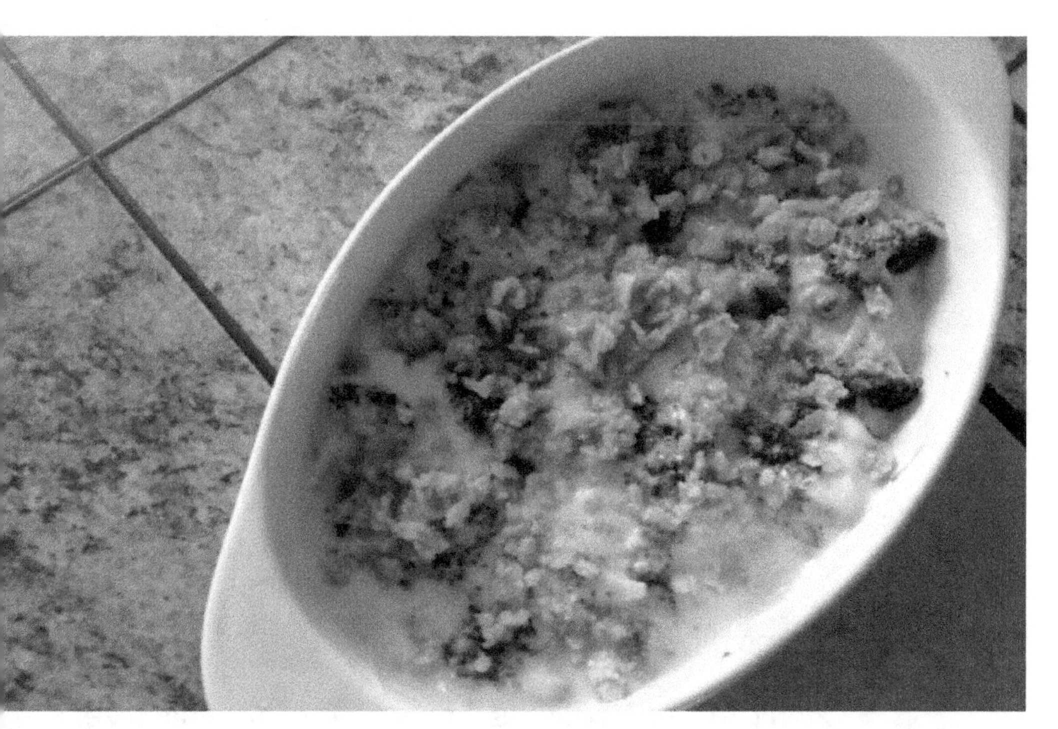

Parmesan Brussels Sprouts

Preparation Time: 5 minutes

Cooking Time: 12 minutes

Serve: 4

Ingredients:

- 1 lb. Brussels sprouts cut stems and halved
- 1 1/2 tbsp. olive oil
- 1/4 cup parmesan cheese, grated
- Pepper
- Salt

Directions:

1. Toss Brussels sprouts, oil, pepper, and salt into the bowl.

2. Transfer Brussels sprouts into the air fryer basket.

3. Place air fryer basket into the oven, and select air fry mode; set Omni to 350 F for 12 minutes. Stir twice.

4. Top with parmesan cheese and serve.

Nutrition:

Calories 114

Fat 7 g

Carbohydrates 10.6 g

Sugar 2.5 g

Protein 5.9 g

Cholesterol 4 mg

Garlicky Cauliflower Florets

Preparation Time: 5 minutes

Cooking Time: 20 minutes

Serve: 4

Ingredients:

- 5 cups cauliflower florets
- 1/2 tsp. cumin powder
- 1/2 tsp. coriander powder
- Six garlic cloves, chopped
- Four tablespoons olive oil
- 1/2 tsp. salt

Directions:

1. Add all ingredients into the large bowl and toss well.

2. Add cauliflower florets into the air fryer basket.

3. Place air fryer basket into the oven, and select air fry mode. Set Omni to 400 F for 20 minutes. Stir twice.

4. Serve and enjoy.

Nutrition:

Calories 159

Fat 14.2 g

Carbohydrates 8.2 g

Sugar 3.1 g

Protein 2.8 g

Cholesterol 0 mg

Flavors Green Beans

Preparation Time: 5 minutes

Cooking Time: 10 minutes

Serve: 2

Ingredients:

- 2 cups green beans
- 1/8 tsp. cayenne pepper
- 1/8 tsp. ground allspice
- 1/4 tsp. ground cinnamon
- 1/2 tsp. dried oregano
- 2 tbsp. olive oil
- 1/4 tsp. ground coriander
- 1/4 tsp. ground cumin
- 1/2 tsp. salt

Directions:

1. Add all ingredients into the mixing bowl and toss well.

2. Spray air fryer basket with cooking spray.

3. Add bowl mixture into the air fryer basket.

4. Place air fryer basket into the oven, and select air fry mode; set Omni to 370 F for 10 minutes.

5. Serve and enjoy.

Nutrition:

Calories 158

Fat 14.3 g

Carbohydrates 8.6 g

Sugar 1.6 g

Protein 2.1 g

Cholesterol 0 mg

Potato Casserole

Preparation Time: 5 minutes

Cooking Time: 35 minutes

Serve: 6

Ingredients:

- Five eggs

- 1/2 cup cheddar cheese, shredded

- Two medium potatoes, diced into 1/2-inch cubes

- One green bell pepper, diced

- One onion, chopped

- 1 tbsp. olive oil

- 3/4 tsp. pepper

- 3/4 tsp. salt

Directions:

1. Spray 9*9-inch casserole dish with cooking spray and set aside.

2. Heat olive oil in a large pan over medium heat.

3. Add onion and sauté for 1 minute. Add potatoes, bell peppers, ½ tsp. Black pepper, and 1.2 tsp. Salt and sauté for 4 minutes more or until onions are softened.

4. Transfer sautéed vegetables to the prepared casserole dish and spread evenly.

5. In a bowl, whisk eggs, and remaining pepper and salt.

6. Pour egg mixture into the casserole dish and sprinkle cheddar cheese on top.

7. Select bake mode and set the Omni to 350 F for 35 minutes. Once the oven beeps, place the casserole dish into the oven.

8. Serve and enjoy.

Nutrition:

Calories 174

Fat 9.2 g

Carbohydrates 14.9 g

Sugar 2.9 g

Protein 8.6 g

Cholesterol 146 mg

48

Zucchini Egg Bake

Preparation Time: 5 minutes

Cooking Time: 30 minutes

Serve: 4

Ingredients:

- Six eggs
- 1/2 tsp. dill
- 1/2 tsp. oregano
- 1/2 tsp. basil
- 1/2 tsp. baking powder
- 1/2 cup almond flour
- 1 cup cheddar cheese, shredded
- 1 cup kale, chopped
- One onion, chopped
- 1 cup zucchini, shredded and squeezed out all liquid
- 1/2 cup milk
- 1/4 tsp. salt

Directions:

1. Grease 9*9-inch baking dish and set aside.

2. In a large bowl, whisk eggs with milk.

3. Add remaining ingredients and stir until well combined.

4. Pour egg mixture into the prepared baking dish.

5. Select bake mode and set the Omni to 375 F for 30 minutes once the oven beeps, place the baking dish into the oven.

6. Serve and enjoy.

Nutrition:

Calories 269

Fat 18.4 g

Carbohydrates 8.9 g

Sugar 3.8 g

Protein 18.3 g

Cholesterol 278 mg

Balsamic Baked Mushrooms

Preparation Time: 5 minutes

Cooking Time: 20 minutes

Serve: 6

Ingredients:

- 1 lb. button mushrooms, scrubbed and stems trimmed
- 2 tbsp. olive oil
- 4 tbsp. balsamic vinegar
- 1/2 tsp. dried basil
- 1/2 tsp. dried oregano
- Three garlic cloves, crushed
- 1/4 tsp. black pepper
- 1 tsp. sea salt

Directions:

1. Spray a cooking pan with cooking spray and set aside.

2. In a large bowl, whisk together vinegar, basil, oregano, garlic, olive oil, pepper, and

salt.

3. Stir in mushrooms and let sit for 15 minutes.

4. Spread mushrooms onto the prepared cooking pan.

5. Select bake mode and set the Omni to 425 F for 20 minutes once the oven beeps, place the cooking pan into the oven.

6. Serve and enjoy.

Nutrition:

Calories 61

Fat 4.9 g

Carbohydrates 3.2 g

Sugar 1.4 g

Protein 2.5 g

Cholesterol 0 mg

Curried Cauliflower

Preparation Time: 10 minutes

Cooking Time: 15 minutes

Serve: 4

Ingredients:

- 2 lbs. cauliflower, cut into florets
- 1 1/2 tsp. curry powder
- 1 tbsp. olive oil
- 1 tbsp. cilantro, chopped
- 2 tsp. fresh lemon juice
- 1 tsp. kosher salt

Directions:

1. Toss cauliflower florets in a large bowl with olive oil.

2. Sprinkle cauliflower florets with curry powder and salt.

3. Spread cauliflower florets onto a cooking pan.

4. Select bake mode and set the Omni to 425 F for 15 minutes once the oven beeps, place the cooking pan into the oven.

5. Return roasted cauliflower florets into the bowl and toss with cilantro and lemon juice.

6. Serve and enjoy.

Nutrition:

Calories 90

Fat 3.9 g

Carbohydrates 12.5 g

Sugar 5.5 g

Protein 4.6 g

Cholesterol 0 mg

Carnitas

Preparation Time: 10 minutes

Cooking Time: 140 minutes

Serving: 4

Ingredients

- 1½ pounds pork shoulder or butt

- 2teaspoons kosher salt

- ½ onion, chopped

- 4cloves garlic, minced

- 1tablespoon vegetable oil

- 1½ cups chicken broth

- ½ teaspoon oregano

- ½ teaspoon chili powder

- ½ teaspoon coriander

- ½ teaspoon cumin

- ½ teaspoon black pepper

- 3bay leaves

- ¼ cup cilantro, chopped

- 1lime, juiced

Directions:

1. Season the pork on all sides with kosher salt.

2. Place pork in a skillet over high heat. Brown all sides.

3. Place pork in the casserole dish.

4. Place chopped onions in the heated skillet and sauté for 3 minutes.

5. Add minced garlic and vegetable oil and sauté for an additional 2 minutes.

6. Add chicken broth, oregano, chili powder, coriander, cumin, black pepper, and bay leaves. Reduce heat to a simmer and cook for 5 minutes.

7. Pour chicken broth mixture into the casserole dish with the pork. Add cilantro and lime juice.

8. Insert the wire rack at a low position in the COSORI Air Fryer Toaster Oven and set the casserole dish on top.

9. Select the Bake function, and then set time to 2 hours 10 minutes and temperature to 350°F. Press Start/Cancel twice to skip preheating and begin baking immediately.

10. Flip the pork with 1 hour left of cook time.

11. Remove when done and serve.

Nutrition:

Calories 583, Total Fat 43g, Carbs 6g, Protein 43g

Greek Lamb Meatballs

Preparation Time: 10minutes

Cooking Time: 12 minutes

Serving: 12

Ingredients:

- 1pound ground lamb
- ½ cup breadcrumbs
- ¼ cup milk
- 2egg yolks
- 1teaspoon ground coriander
- 1teaspoon ground cumin
- 3garlic cloves, minced
- 1teaspoon dried oregano
- ½ teaspoon salt
- ½ teaspoon black pepper
- 1lemon juiced and zested
- ¼ cup fresh parsley, chopped
- ½ cup crumbled feta cheese

- Olive oil, for shaping

- Tzatziki, for dipping

Directions:

1. Combine all ingredients except olive oil in a large mixing bowl and mix until fully incorporated.

2. Form 12 meatballs, about 2 ounces each. Use olive oil on your hands, so they don't stick to the meatballs. Set aside.

3. Select the Broil function on the COSORI Air Fryer Toaster Oven, set time to 12 minutes, then press Start/Cancel to preheat.

4. Place the meatballs on the food tray, then insert the tray at the top position in the preheated air fryer toaster oven. Press Start/Cancel.

5. Take out the meatballs when done and serve with a side of tzatziki.

Nutrition:

Calories 129, Total Fat 6.4g, Total Carbs 4.9g, Protein 12.9g

Sesame Ginger Pork Meatballs

Preparation Time: 10 minutes

Cooking Time: 12 minutes

Serving: 12

Ingredients:

- 1pound ground pork

- 3shiitake mushrooms, finely chopped

- 2scallions, finely chopped

- 2cabbage leaves, finely chopped

- 1½-inch-thick piece of ginger, grated

- 1½ teaspoons sesame oil

- 1tablespoon soy sauce

- ¾ teaspoon salt

- 1teaspoon sugar

- ¼ teaspoon black pepper

- 1½ tablespoons cornstarch

- Canola oil, for shaping

- Sesame seeds, for garnish

Directions:

1. Mix the pork, mushrooms, scallions, cabbage, ginger, sesame oil, soy sauce, salt, sugar, black pepper, and cornstarch until well combined.

2. Form 12 meatballs, about 2 ounces each. Use canola oil on your hands, so they don't stick to the meatballs. Set aside.

3. Select the Broil function on the COSORI Air Fryer Toaster Oven, set time to 10 minutes, and press Start/Cancel to preheat.

4. Place the meatballs on the food tray, then insert the tray at the top position in the preheated air fryer toaster oven. Press Start/Cancel.

5. Remove when done and garnish with sesame seeds, then serve.

Nutrition:

Calories 110, Total Fat 4.6g, Total Carbs 6.7g, Protein 10.4g

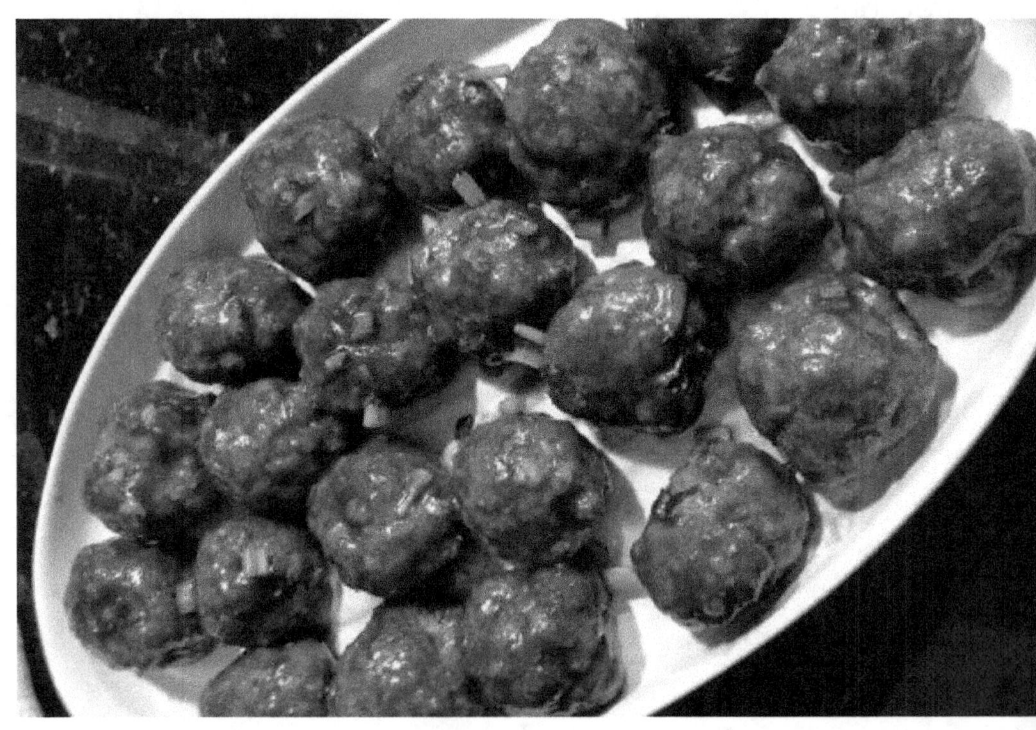

Chili Beef Skewers

Preparation Time: 10 minutes

Cooking Time: 130 minutes

Serving: 2

Ingredients:

- 1ribeye steak (1 pound), cut into 2-inch cubes

- ¼ cup olive oil

- 1tablespoon chili powder

- 2teaspoons salt

- 1teaspoon cumin

- 1teaspoon oregano

- ½ teaspoon garlic powder

- ½ teaspoon black pepper

- 1lime, juiced

- 1red bell pepper, cut into 2-inch squares

- ½ onion, cut into 2-inch squares

Directions:

1. Combine steak, olive oil, chili powder, salt, cumin, oregano, garlic powder, black pepper, and lime juice in a plastic resealable bag.

2. Shake well and marinate for 2 hours in the fridge.

3. Skewer the meat, inserting red bell pepper and onion between each piece of steak. Set aside.

4. Select the Broil function on the COSORI Air Fryer Toaster Oven, set time to 10 minutes, then press Start/Cancel to preheat.

5. Place skewers on the food tray, then insert the tray at the top position in the preheated air fryer toaster oven. Press Start/Cancel.

6. Remove when done and serve.

Nutrition:

Calories 1352, Total Fat 100g, Total Carbs 18g, Protein 95g

Chipotle Pork Tenderloin Roast

Preparation Time: 40 minutes

Cooking Time: 30 minutes

Serving: 4

Ingredients:

- 1pound pork tenderloin, whole

- 1can or 7 ounces chipotle peppers in adobo sauce

- 1teaspoon salt

- 1teaspoon black pepper

- ½ red or white onion, sliced

- 4cloves garlic, whole

- 2tablespoons olive oil

Directions:

1. Mix the pork tenderloin, chipotle peppers, salt, and black pepper in a large plastic resealable bag.

2. Marinate for 30 minutes.

3. Select the Roast function on the COSORI Air Fryer Toaster Oven, set time to 30 minutes and temperature to 400°F, then press Start/Cancel to preheat.

4. Place a layer of aluminum foil on the food tray and set the pork tenderloin on top.

5. Place onion and garlic around the tenderloin and drizzle olive oil over the onion.

6. Insert food tray at a low position in the preheated air fryer toaster oven. Press Start/Cancel.

7. Remove when done and allow cooling for 5 minutes.

8. Spoon onions and garlic over the tenderloin and serve.

Nutrition:

Calories 234, Total Fat 11.3g, Total Carbs 2.7g, Protein 30.3g

Italian Ribeye Steak

Preparation Time: 10 minutes

Cooking Time: 15 minutes

Serving: 2-3

Ingredients:

- 1ribeye steak (12-14 ounces)
    - ¼ cup flat-leaf parsley, minced
- ¼ cup basil, minced
- 3cloves garlic, minced
- 3tablespoons olive oil
- ½ lemon, juiced
- ¾ teaspoon coarse black pepper, divided
- 1¼ teaspoons kosher salt, divided

Directions:

1. Mix parsley, basil, garlic, olive oil, lemon juice, ¼ teaspoon black pepper, and ¼ teaspoon salt in a bowl. Refrigerate until ready to use.

2. Sprinkle the remaining salt and pepper on both sides of the rib eye steak.

3. Select the Broil function on the COSORI Air Fryer Toaster Oven, set the temperature to

450°F, then press Start/Cancel to preheat.

4. Place the steak on the food tray, insert the tray at the top position in the preheated air fryer toaster oven, and then press Start/Cancel.

5. Move steak to a plate when done, remix the parsley mixture, and spoon over steak.

6. Allow the steak to rest for 3 minutes and then serve.

Nutrition:

Calories 856, Total Fat 64g, Total Carbs 7.1g, Protein 62.9g

Lamb Gyro

Preparation Time: 10 minutes

Cooking Time: 25 minutes

Serving: 4

Ingredients:

- 1pound ground lamb
- ¼ red onion, minced
- ¼ cup mint, minced
- ¼ cup parsley, minced
- 2cloves garlic, minced
- ½ teaspoon salt
- ⅛ teaspoon rosemary
- ½ teaspoon black pepper
- 4slices pita bread
- ¾ cup hummus
- 1cup romaine lettuce, shredded
- ½ onion sliced
- 1Roma tomato, diced

- ½ cucumber, skinned and thinly sliced

- 12mint leaves, minced

- Tzatziki sauce, to taste

Directions:

1. Mix ground lamb, red onion, mint, parsley, garlic, salt, rosemary, and black pepper until fully incorporated.

2. Select the Broil function on the COSORI Air Fryer Toaster Oven, set time to 25 minutes and temperature to 450°F, then press Start/Cancel to preheat.

3. Line the food tray with parchment paper and place the ground lamb on top, shaping it into a patty 1-inch-thick and 6 inches in diameter.

4. Insert the food tray at the top position in the preheated air fryer toaster oven, then press Start/Cancel.

5. Remove when done and cut into thin slices.

6. Assemble each gyro starting with pita bread, then hummus, lamb meat, lettuce, onion, tomato, cucumber, and mint leaves, drizzle with tzatziki.

7. Serve immediately.

Nutrition:

Calories 409, Total Fat 14.6g, Total Carbs 29.9g, Protein 39.4g

Sausage Hot Pot

Preparation Time: 10 minutes

Cooking Time: 65 minutes

Serving: 2

Ingredients:

- 1tablespoon vegetable oil
- 5fresh brat sausages or mild Italian sausages
- 2tablespoons unsalted butter
- ¼ teaspoon kosher salt
- ¼ teaspoon black pepper
- 5sprigs thyme
- 1whole onion, sliced
- 12cremini mushrooms, sliced
- ½ cup red wine
- 1cup beef broth
- 1tablespoon parsley, chopped

Directions:

1. Insert the wire rack at mid-position in the COSORI Air Fryer Toaster Oven. Select the Broil function, set timer to 40 minutes and temperature to 350°F, then press Start/Cancel to preheat.

2. Pour vegetable oil in a skillet over high heat and brown sausages on both sides for 10 minutes and then set aside.

3. Place butter, salt, black pepper, thyme, sliced onion, and mushrooms in the same skillet, reduce heat to medium, and sauté for 10 minutes or until onions are soft.

4. Pour red wine and beef broth into the skillet and simmer for 5 minutes.

5. Pour the onion mixture and broth into the casserole dish, and then place the sausages so that they're half immersed.

6. Place the casserole dish on the wire rack in the preheated air fryer toaster oven, then press Start/Cancel.

7. Remove casserole dish when done, garnish with parsley, and then serve.

Nutrition:

Calories 716, Total Fat 26.4g, Total Carbs 91.8g, Protein 27.4g

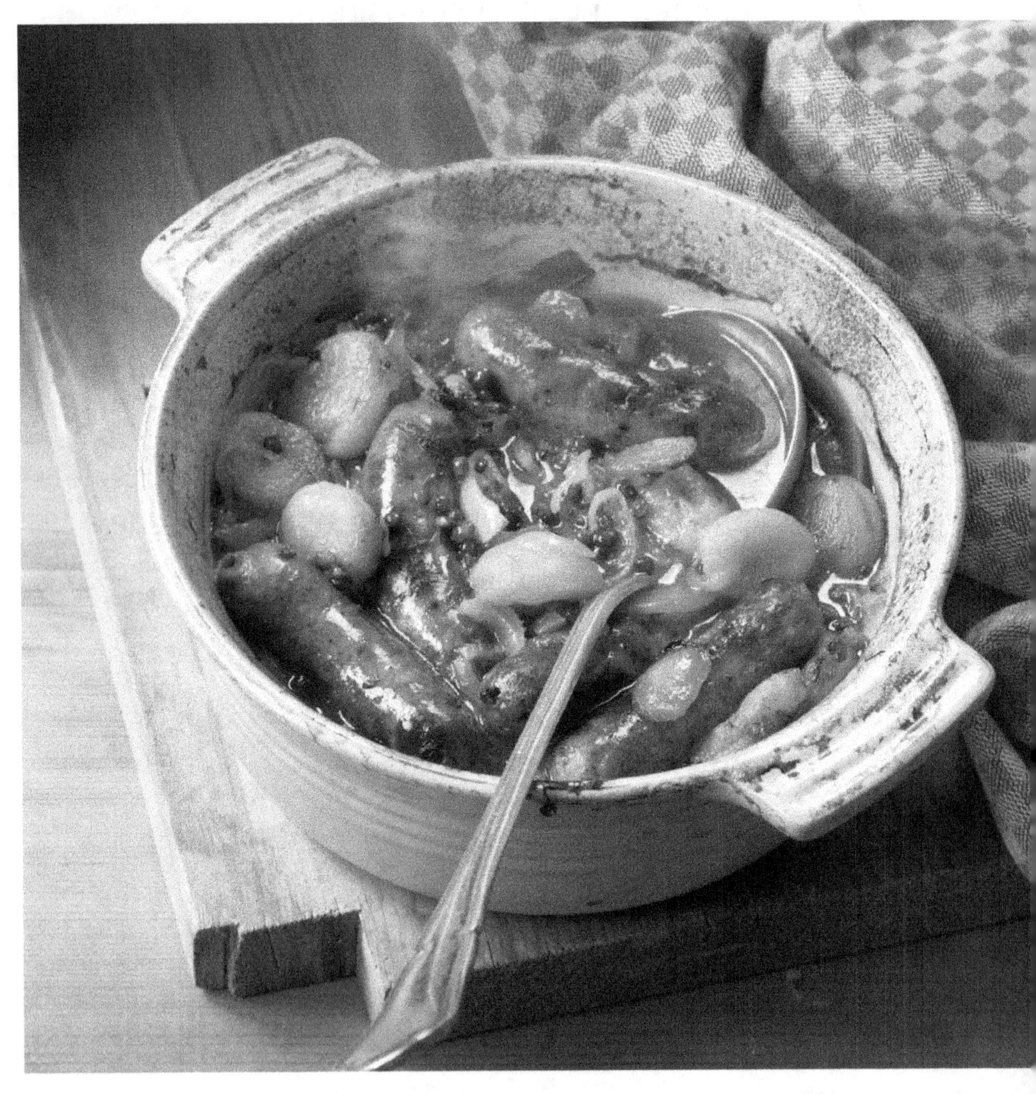

Roast Beef

Preparation Time: 15 minutes

Cooking Time: 60 minutes

Serving: 6

Ingredients:

- 1round roast (3 pounds)
  - 1teaspoon salt

- ½ teaspoon paprika
- ½ teaspoon garlic powder
- ½ teaspoon black pepper
- 1tablespoon olive oil
- 1tablespoon Dijon mustard

Directions:

1. Mix salt, paprika, garlic powder, black pepper, olive oil, and Dijon mustard in a small bowl.

2. Select the Roast function on the COSORI Air Fryer Toaster Oven, set time to 1 hour and temperature to 380°F, then press Start/Cancel to preheat.

3. Rub the round roast with the Dijon mixture until fully covered.

4. Place round roast on the food tray and insert the food tray at a low position in the preheated air fryer toaster oven. Press Start/Cancel.

5. Remove roast when done and let it rest for 10 minutes, then slice and serve.

Nutrition:

Calories 138, Total Fat 9.6g, Total Carbs 0.56g, Protein 12.4g

Air Fried Brussels Sprouts

Preparation Time: 5 minutes

Cooking time: 10 minutes

Servings: 1

Ingredients

- 1 pound (454 g) Brussels sprouts

- One tablespoon coconut oil, melted

- One tablespoon unsalted butter, melted

Directions

1. Preheat the air fryer oven to 400ºF (204ºC).

2. Prepare the Brussels sprouts by halving them, discarding any loose leaves.

3. Combine with the melted coconut oil and transfer to the air fryer basket.

4. Place the air fryer basket onto the baking pan and slide into Rack Position 2, select Air Fry, and set time to 10 minutes, shaking the basket once cooking. The sprouts are ready when they are partially caramelized.

5. Remove from the oven and serve with a topping of melted butter.

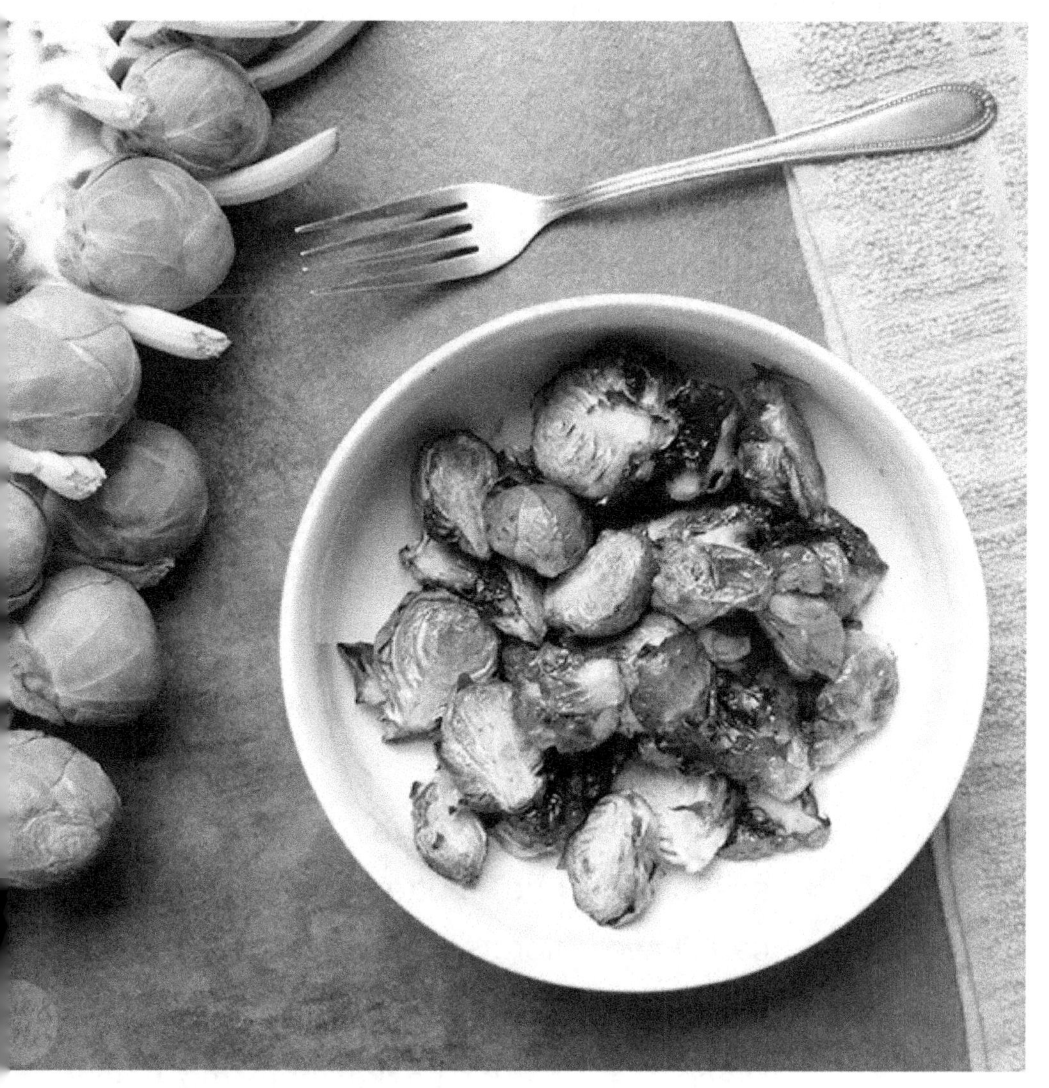

Simple Buffalo Cauliflower

Preparation Time: 5 minutes

Cooking time: 5 minutes

Servings: 1

Ingredients

- ½ packet dry ranch seasoning
- Two tablespoons salted butter, melted
- 1 cup cauliflower florets
- ¼ cup buffalo sauce

Directions

1. Preheat the air fryer oven to 400ºF (204ºC).

2. In a bowl, combine the dry ranch seasoning and butter. Toss with the cauliflower florets to coat and transfer them to the air fryer basket.

3. Place the air fryer basket onto the baking pan and slide into Rack Position 2; select Air Fry, and set time to 5 minutes, shaking

the basket occasionally to ensure the florets cook evenly.

4. Remove the cauliflower and place it on a platter. Pour the buffalo sauce over it and serve warm.

Crispy Jicama Fries

Preparation Time: 5 minutes

Cooking time: 20 minutes

Servings: 1

Ingredients

- One small jicama, peeled
- ¼ teaspoon onion powder
- ¾ teaspoon chili powder
- ¼ teaspoon garlic powder
- ¼ teaspoon ground black pepper

Directions

1. Preheat the air fryer oven to 350ºF (177ºC).

2. To make the fries, cut the jicama into matchsticks of the desired thickness.

3. In a bowl, toss them with the onion powder, chili powder, garlic powder, and black pepper to coat. Transfer the fries into the air fryer basket.

4. Place the air fryer basket onto the baking pan and slide into Rack Position 2, select Air Fry, and set time to 20 minutes, giving the basket an occasional shake throughout the cooking process. The fries are ready when they are hot and golden.

5. Serve immediately.

Zucchini Balls

Preparation Time: 5 minutes

Cooking time: 10 minutes

Servings: 4

Ingredients

- Four zucchinis
- One egg
- ½ cup grated Parmesan cheese
- One tablespoon Italian herbs
- 1 cup grated coconut

Directions

1. Thinly grate the zucchinis and dry with cheesecloth, ensuring to remove all the moisture.

2. In a bowl, combine the zucchinis with the egg, Parmesan, Italian herbs, and grated coconut, mixing well to incorporate everything. Using the hands, mold the mixture into balls.

3. Preheat the air fryer oven to 400ºF (204ºC).

4. Lay the zucchini balls in the air fryer basket.

5. Place the air fryer basket onto the baking pan and slide into Rack Position 2, select Air Fry, and set time to 10 minutes.

6. Serve hot.

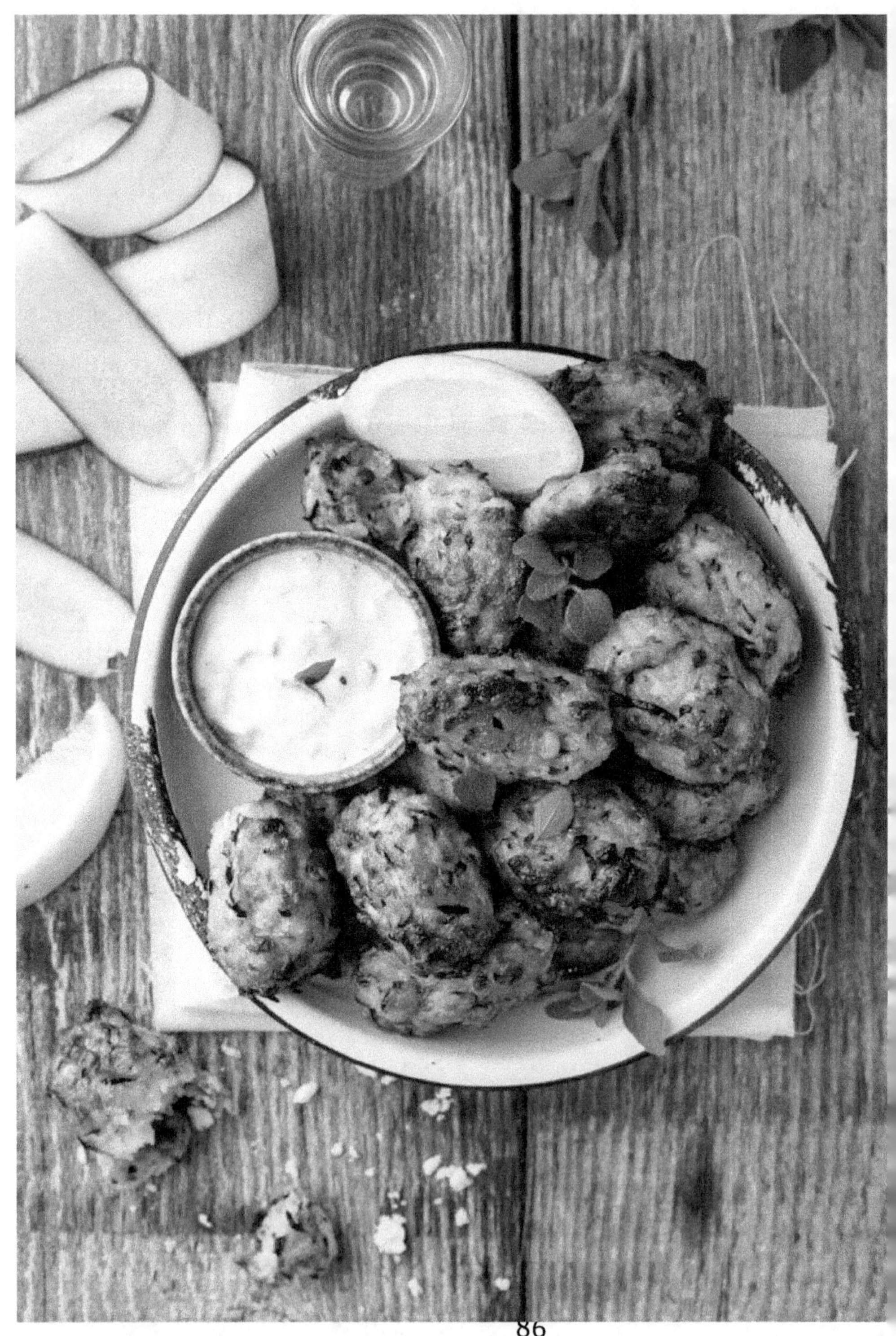

Cheesy Potatoes And Asparagus 10

Preparation Time: 5 minutes

Cooking time: 23 minutes

Servings: 4

Ingredients

- Four medium potatoes

- One bunch asparagus

- ⅓ cup cottage cheese

- ⅓ cup low-fat crème Fraiche

- One tablespoon wholegrain mustard

- Salt and pepper, to taste

- Cooking spray

Directions

1. Preheat the air fryer oven to 390ºF (199ºC). Spritz the air fryer basket with cooking spray.

2. Place the potatoes in the basket. Place the air fryer basket onto the baking pan and slide into Rack Position 2, select Air Fry, and set time to 20 minutes.

3. Meanwhile, boil the asparagus in salted water for 3 minutes.

4. Remove the potatoes and mash them with the rest of the ingredients. Sprinkle with salt and pepper.

5. Serve immediately.

Saltine Wax Beans

Preparation Time: 10 minutes

Cooking time: 7 minutes

Servings: 4

Ingredients:

- ½ cup flour
- One teaspoon smoky chipotle powder
- ½ teaspoon ground black pepper
- One teaspoon sea salt flakes
- Two eggs, beaten
- ½ cup crushed saltines
- 10 ounces (283 g) wax beans
- Cooking spray

Directions:

1. Preheat the air fryer oven to 360ºF (182ºC).

2. Combine all ingredients the flour, chipotle powder, black pepper, and salt in a bowl.

3. In the second bowl, put the two beaten eggs.

4. Provide another bowl of crushed saltines.

5. Wash the beans with cold water and discard any tough strings.

6. Coat the beans with the flour mixture before dipping them into the beaten egg. Cover them with the crushed saltines.

7. Spritz the beans with cooking spray, and then transfer to the air fryer basket.

8. Place the air fryer basket onto the baking pan and slide into Rack Position 2, select Air Fry, and set time to 4 minutes.

9. Give the air fryer basket a fair shake and continue to air fry for 3 minutes. Serve hot.

Potato With Creamy Cheese

Preparation Time: 5minutes

Cooking time: 15 minutes

Servings: 2

Ingredients:

- Two medium potatoes

- One teaspoon butter

- Three tablespoons sour cream

- One teaspoon chives

- 1½ tablespoons grated Parmesan cheese

Directions:

1. Preheat the air fryer oven to 350ºF (177ºC).

2. Pierce the potatoes with a fork and boil them in water until they are cooked. Transfer to the air fryer basket.

3. Place the air fryer basket onto the baking pan and slide into Rack Position 2, select Air Fry, and set time to 15 minutes.

4. In the meantime, combine the sour cream, cheese, and chives in a bowl. Cut the potatoes halfway to open them up and fill with the butter and sour cream mixture.

5. Serve immediately.

Easy Rosemary Green Beans

Preparation Time: 5 minutes

Cooking time: 5minutes

Servings: 1

Ingredients:

- One tablespoon butter, melted

- Two tablespoons rosemary

- ½ teaspoon salt

- Three cloves garlic, minced

- ¾ cup chopped green beans

Directions:

1. Preheat the air fryer oven to 390ºF (199ºC).

2. Combine the melted butter with the rosemary, salt, and minced garlic. Toss in the green beans, coating them well. Transfer to the air fryer basket.

3. Place the air fryer basket onto the baking pan and slide into Rack Position 2, select

Air Fry, and set time to 5 minutes.

4. Serve immediately.

Garlic Eggplant Slices

Preparation Time: 5 minutes

Cooking time: 15 minutes

Servings: 1

Ingredients:

- One large eggplant, sliced
- Two tablespoons olive oil
- ¼ teaspoon salt
- ½ teaspoon garlic powder

Directions:

1. Preheat the air fryer oven to 390ºF (199ºC).

2. Toss the eggplant slices with the olive oil, salt, and garlic powder in a mixing bowl until evenly coated.

3. Put the slices in the air fryer basket. Place the air fryer basket onto the baking pan and slide into Rack Position 2, select Air Fry, and set time to 15 minutes.

4. Serve immediately.

Herbed Radishes

Preparation Time: 5 minutes

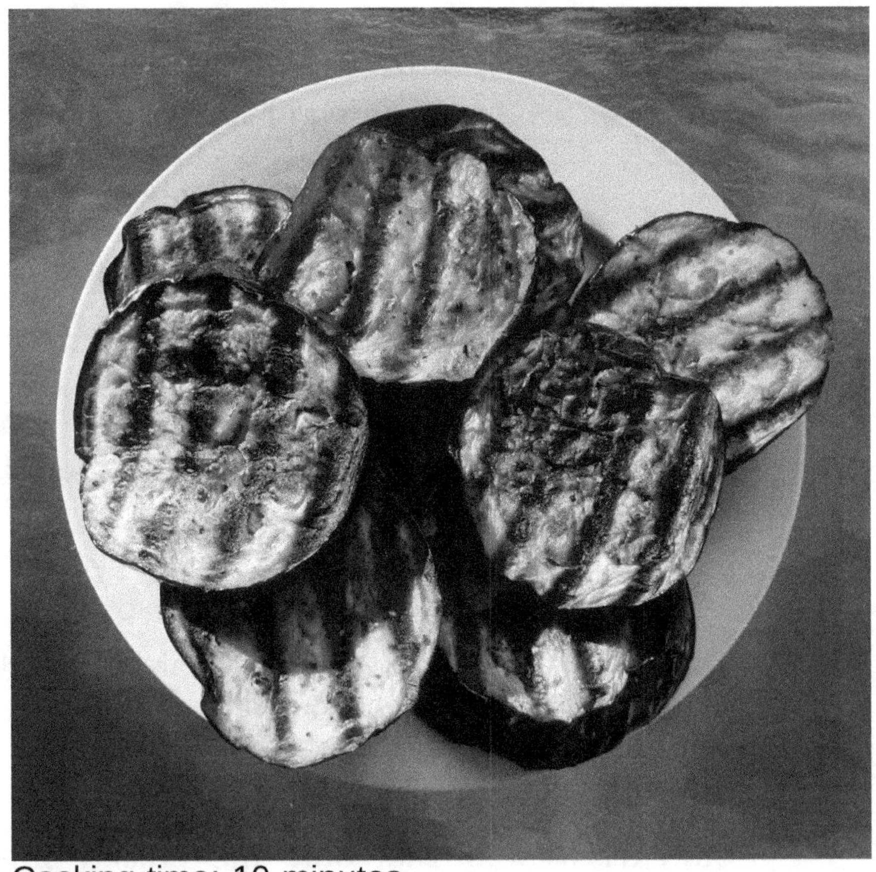

Cooking time: 10 minutes

Servings: 2

Ingredients:

- 1 pound (454 g) radishes

- Two tablespoons unsalted butter, melted

- ¼ teaspoon dried oregano

- ½ teaspoon dried parsley

- ½ teaspoon garlic powder

Directions:

1. Preheat the air fryer oven to 350ºF (177ºC).

2. Prepare the radishes by cutting off their tops and bottoms and quartering them.

3. In a bowl, combine the butter, dried oregano, dried parsley, and garlic powder. Toss with the radishes to coat. Transfer the radishes to the air fryer basket.

4. Place the air fryer basket onto the baking pan and slide into Rack Position 2, select Air Fry, and set time to 10 minutes. Shake the basket halfway through. The radishes are ready when they turn brown.

5. Serve immediately.

Sesame Taj Tofu

Preparation Time: 5 minutes

Cooking time: 25 minutes

Servings: 4

Ingredients:

- One block firm tofu pressed and cut into 1-inch thick cubes

- Two tablespoons soy sauce

- Two teaspoons toasted sesame seeds

- One teaspoon rice vinegar

- One tablespoon cornstarch

Directions:

1. Preheat the air fryer oven to 400ºF (204ºC).

2. Add the tofu, soy sauce, sesame seeds, and rice vinegar in a bowl and mix well to coat the tofu cubes. Then cover the tofu in cornstarch and put it in the air fryer basket.

3. Place the air fryer basket onto the baking pan and slide into Rack Position 2, select Air Fry, and set time to 25 minutes, giving the basket a shake at 5-minute intervals to ensure the tofu cooks evenly.

4. Serve immediately.

Chili Fingerling Potatoes

Preparation Time: 10 minutes

Cooking time: 16 minutes

Servings: 4

Ingredients:

- 1 pound (454 g) fingerling potatoes, rinsed and cut into wedges
- One teaspoon olive oil
- One teaspoon salt
- One teaspoon black pepper
- One teaspoon cayenne pepper
- One teaspoon nutritional yeast
- ½ teaspoon garlic powder

Directions:

1. Preheat the air fryer oven to 400ºF (204ºC).

2. Coat the potatoes with the rest of the ingredients. Transfer to the air fryer basket.

3. Place the air fryer basket onto the baking pan and slide into Rack Position 2, select Air Fry, and set time to 16 minutes, shaking the basket halfway through the cooking time.

4. Serve immediately.

Sweet And Sour Tofu

Preparation Time: 15 minutes

Cooking time: 20 minutes

Servings: 2

Ingredients:

- Two teaspoons apple cider vinegar

- One tablespoon sugar

- One tablespoon soy sauce

- Three teaspoons lime juice

- One teaspoon ground ginger

- One teaspoon garlic powder

- ½ block firm tofu pressed to remove excess liquid and cut into cubes

- One teaspoon cornstarch

- Two green onions, chopped

- Toasted sesame seeds, for garnish

Directions:

1. In a bowl, thoroughly combine the apple cider vinegar, sugar, soy sauce, lime juice, ground ginger, and garlic powder.

2. Cover the tofu with this mixture and leave to marinate for at least 30 minutes.

3. Preheat the air fryer oven to 400ºF (204ºC).

4. Transfer the tofu to the air fryer basket, keeping any excess marinade for the sauce.

5. Place the air fryer basket onto the baking pan and slide into Rack Position 2. Select Air Fry and set time to 20 minutes, or until crispy.

6. In the meantime, thicken the sauce with the cornstarch over medium-low heat.

7. Serve the cooked tofu with the sauce, green onions, and sesame seeds.

Easy Potato Croquettes

Preparation Time: 15minutes

Cooking Time: 15 minutes

Serving: 10

Ingredients:

- ¼ cup nutritional yeast
- 2 cups boiled potatoes, mashed
- One flax egg
- One tablespoon flour
- Two tablespoons chopped chives
- Salt and ground black pepper, to taste
- Two tablespoons vegetable oil
- ¼ cup bread crumbs

Directions:

1. Preheat the air fryer oven to 400ºF (204ºC).

2. In a bowl, combine the nutritional yeast, potatoes, flax egg, flour, and chives.

Sprinkle with salt and pepper as desired.

3. In a separate bowl, mix the vegetable oil and bread crumbs to achieve a crumbly consistency.

4. Shape the potato mixture into small balls and dip each one into the bread crumb mixture. Put the croquettes in the air fryer basket.

5. Place the air fryer basket onto the baking pan and slide into Rack Position 2, select Air Fry, and set time to 15 minutes, ensuring the croquettes turn golden brown.

6. Serve immediately.

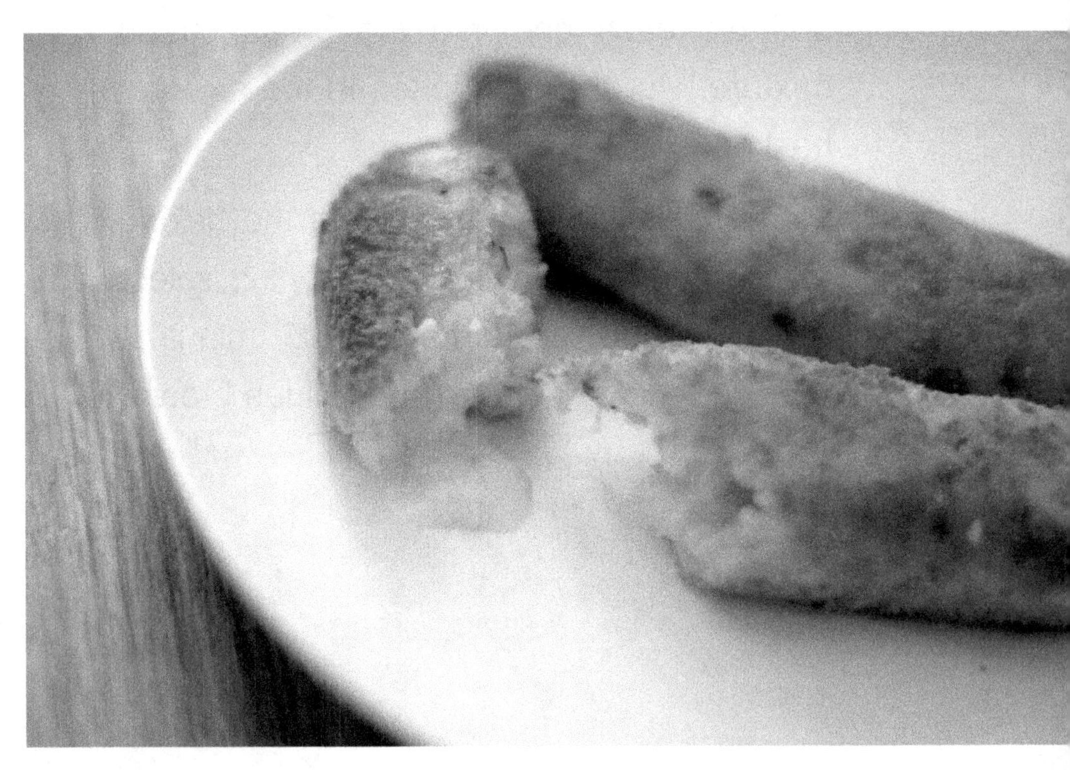